EASY WAYS TO MAINTAIN YOUR IDEAL BODY MASS INDEX
by Oswin Dacosta
www.losingbellyfatmission.com
www.achieveitforyou.com

Legal & Disclaimer

Legal & Disclaimer

The information contained in this book is not designed to replace or take the place of any form of medicine or professional medical advice. The information in this book has been provided for educational and entertainment purposes only.

The information contained in this book has been compiled from sources deemed reliable, and it is accurate to the best of the Author's knowledge; however, the Author cannot guarantee its accuracy and validity and cannot be held liable for any errors or omissions. Changes are periodically made to this book. You must consult your doctor or get professional medical advice before using any of the suggested remedies, techniques, or information in this book.

Upon using the information contained in this book, you agree to hold harmless the Author from and against any damages, costs, and expenses, including any legal fees potentially resulting from the application of any of the information provided by this guide. This disclaimer applies to any damages or injury caused by the use and application, whether directly or indirectly, of any advice or information presented, whether for breach of contract, tort, negligence, personal injury, criminal intent, or under any other cause of action.

You agree to accept all risks of using the information presented inside this book. You need to consult a professional medical practitioner in order to ensure you are both able and healthy enough to participate in this program.

Table of Contents

1. INTRODUCTION

A COMPLETE GUIDE TO MAINTAINING A PERFECT PHYSIQUE

QUICK AND SAFE TACTICS FOR WEIGHTLOSS

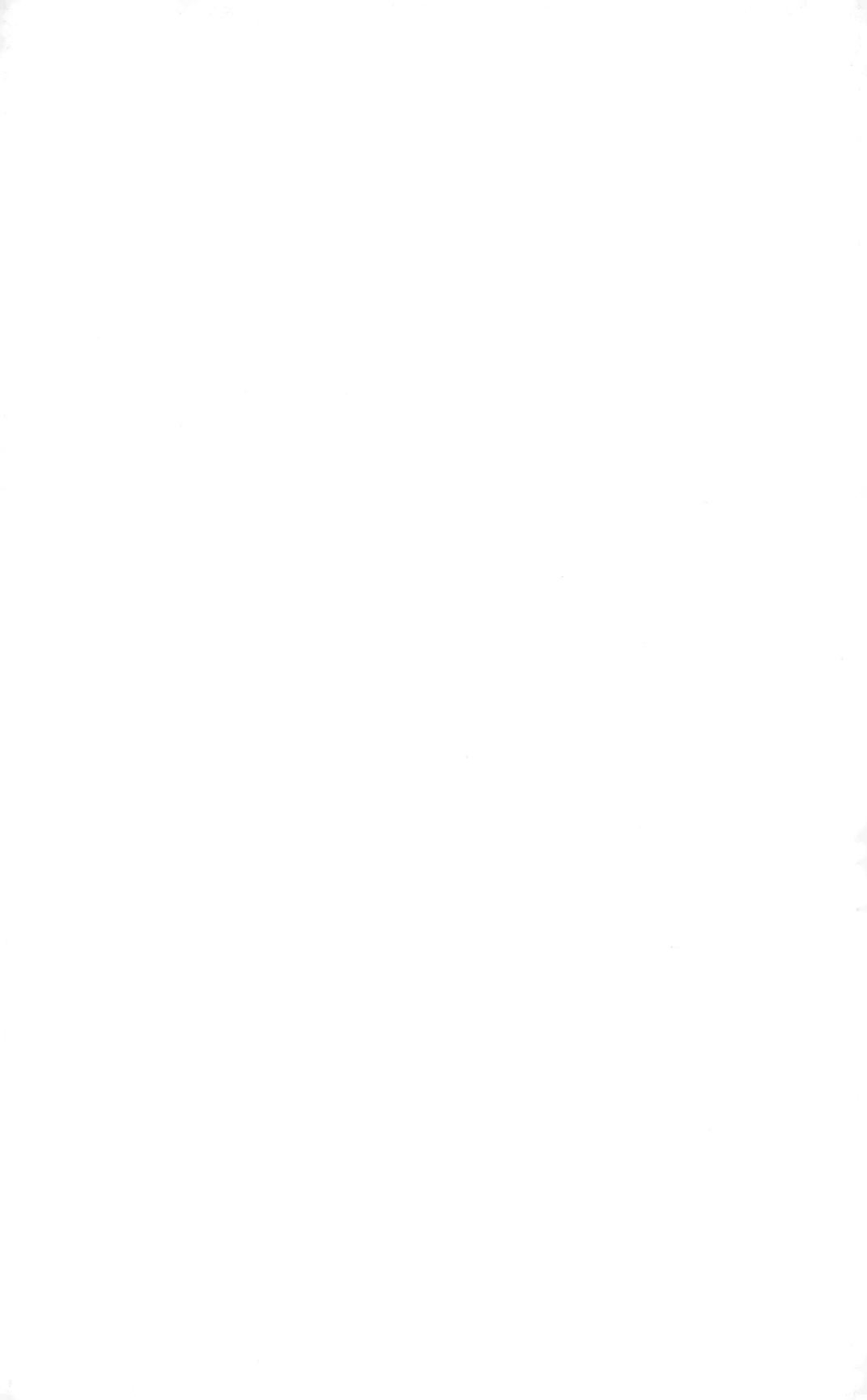

Obesity has become a global problem now-a-days. It has spread like an epidemic all over the world. More than 1.5 billion people are suffering from obesity worldwide. Moreover, one third and above of adults in the US are obese. The main reason for such a widespread condition is unhealthy lifestyle and food. Having a fit body is considered an unachievable dream by many among us. Why it is so important to us to have a fit body? Having a fit body not only gives us confidence in every aspect of our lives, but also provides the groundwork for a lifestyle, which keeps most of lifestyle related ailments at a distance from us. Some people believe that having a fit body or fat body only depends on luck and is granted to us. Although this theory has some scientific base in the form of fast and slow metabolism individuals, but it is not entirely true. Fitness and good physique is not a state that is achieved, but rather it is a lifestyle that we have to live continuously. This might seem daunting that we have to work to be fit every day, but if you really think about it, it's the life you will be living and believe me that it will not be that hard once you are motivated to achieve a healthy and fit physique. It will be just like living a normal life, but making it better and healthier, and will only be a matter of time that you will not even feel like you are working for it. With time, it will be like a normal routine for you.

keeps most of lifestyle related ailments at a distance from us. Some people believe that having a fit body or fat body only depends on luck and is granted to us. Although this theory has some scientific base in the form of fast and slow metabolism individuals, but it is not entirely true. Fitness and good physique is not a state that is achieved, but rather it is a lifestyle that we have to live continuously. This might seem daunting that we have to work to be fit every day, but if you really think about it, it's the life you will be living and believe me that it will not be that hard once you are motivated to achieve a healthy and fit physique. It will be just like living a normal life, but making it better and healthier, and will only be a matter of time that you will not even feel like you are working for it. With time, it will be like a normal routine for you.

Maintaining a healthy weight is important for overall health. It helps prevent many prevalent disease like hypertension, diabetes, cardiovascular problems, gallstones and even certain cancers. Moreover, having a healthy weight gives you confidence and makes you feel good about yourself. Life with good physique will be comparatively more joyful for every human being on this planet.

It is absolutely possible to lose weight and reach an ideal mass; don't find an excuse that it is not impossible so that you may not have to work for it. It won't happen in the blink of an eye, but it will happen eventually. Reaching and maintaining an ideal weight is a harmony between food and activity. You will need some balance between intake and utilization of food and some attitude, motivation and self-control. The key is not some changes in your diet for a short span of time, but you have to make changes in your lifestyle, including healthy eating, regular physical activity and a balance between intake and consumption of calories.

Body Mass Index
What is obesity and overweight? Overweight is having extra body weight from muscle, fat or bone. Obesity is having a high amount of extra body fat. Body mass index is a useful measure of obesity and fitness. Although 'weight' alone can also be used as a unit for those who are trying to maintain a better physical health, but BMI (Body Mass Index) is a better alternative to measuring only weight as it also includes the measures of ones height.

How to calculate BMI
BMI can easily be calculated by the following simple formula.
Your weight (pounds) times 703, divided by the square of your height in inches.
Example:
Weight 195 pounds.
Height 6 ft. (72 inches)
$72^2 = 5184$
195 x 703 = 137085
137085 divided by 5184 = BMI 26.44
According to the most of the health authorities, the following standards are customary.
People with a BMI below **18.5** are considered as underweight.
A BMI of between **18.5 and 25** is ideal.
Individual with a BMI in-between the range **25 and 30** is categorized to be overweight.
A person with a BMI over **30** is obese.
BMI should not be taken as a universal unit in fitness as it has some flaws too, but it gives a pretty good idea of what is present and what should be the target.

2. The Main Factors that Cause Obesity

Chapter 2: The Main Factors that Cause Obesity

Obesity is defined as the abnormal gain of weight due to the accumulation of the fats in the body. A person is called obese when he gains weight that is greater than the standard range with respect to his height. Of course, this is not a healthy condition for anyone, and is among the major concerns now-a-days worldwide as it may lead to many other diseases and health problems.

The standard range that shows a standard measure of weight-for-height is called as BMI (Body Mass Index). As described before, if BMI of a person is calculated to be 30 or above, the person is called obese. The normal range for BMI is 25 and people falling within this range, are said to have normal weight to height ratio. So, you can easily determine whether you are having a normal physique or slowly inclining towards obesity. World Health Organization concluded that obesity has nearly doubled in the past 30 years and is triggered by a number of factors. The 2008 statistics clearly shows that more than 500 million people are obese, among which, 300 million are women and 200 million men.

Here are the main factors which are concerned as the potential triggers of obesity.

1.

Improper Diet Intake

The foremost reason behind obesity is none other than an improper diet. Life has become so busy and hectic for everyone these days. The work schedules do not allow to eat healthier as everyone is in rush for the work and finds it easier to grab a pack of fast food in lunch or dinner without thinking of the consequences. Fast food is usually rich of too many calories, which adds more fat to your body, and turns your body into improper mass. Poor diet and poor lifestyle leads to the development of obesity with time. The poor diet may contain the following, which must be avoided and replaced with healthy, full of vitamins and minerals rich food.

- Processed food with large amounts of fats and sugar should be avoided and replaced with fresh cooked vegetables.
- Alcohol intake leads to accumulation of a large amount of fats as alcohol is rich in calories, thus increase the body weight abnormally.
- Eating desserts after every meal leads to obesity as desserts have a lot of sugar.
- Eating more than required also makes your body save fats and turns your body out of shape.
- Eating junk food is one of the basic potential triggers of obesity.

For enjoying a healthy and diseases-free life, it is important to avoid all the above habits, and adapt healthy eating practice. For maintaining a normal health, it is necessary to take 2000 to 2500 calories per day. People who take more than this amount of calories become obese as body saves all the extra calories in the form of fats.

2. Lack of Physical Activity and Inactive and Sedentary Lifestyle

The second most important factor that is responsible to trigger obesity is the lack of exercise. Generally, people consume a lot of calories and are unable to burn them properly because of the lack of activity. So, these calories ultimately get stored in the body as fats and this storage of fats leads to obesity with time.

People who work in offices rarely do any physical activity. They need to work all day in a sitting posture, which is one of the main causes of storage of the calories they consume. If a person is not doing any regular exercise, nor he prefers walking or cycling over riding the car or motorbike, he is not doing any physical activity and may develop obesity with time.

3. Role of Genetics in obesity

The third factor which is involved in the development of obesity in most of the people is the genetics. Of course, genes are responsible to decide for us. Certain genes are triggered with specific age and environmental factors, when they are already present. It means that the chances of development of obesity in the child of obese parents are more as compared to the child who has lean parents. But, this does not depend entirely on genetics. The researches have proved that the genes for obesity are only triggered when the environmental factors are favorable for their expression, and the environmental factors here are no other than the eating habits. Poor eating habits may develop the disease in the child of obese parents, but, may not develop it in the child of lean parents. So, when it's in your genes, you have to be more concerned and careful with your diet and eating habits to avoiding building up extra body mass.

4. Contribution of Medicines and certain Ailments in development of Obesity

Researches have brought many medicines and ailments into concern that are responsible in the development of obesity. Following are a few examples.

Hypothyroidism

It is the lack of the proper activity of the thyroid gland, which leads to the deficient production of thyroid hormone. In this condition, it is noticed that the body become abnormally large due to the improper regulation of the calories.

Cushing syndrome

It is the syndrome associated with the overproduction of steroid hormones, thus making the diseased person obese.

Medication

There are certain medicines that are actively involved in causing obesity, which include the medicines for diabetes, epilepsy, antidepressants, corticosteroids, drugs taken for treatment of schizophrenia, etc. All these medicines intake contribute to weight gain, leading to obesity with time.

5. Smoking

Obesity can also be developed in response to quitting smoking. In this condition, weight is gained as a side effect for the stoppage of smoking, and person may develop obesity. There are two reasons behind this weight gain. First is the sensation of taste. As it become better for all the foods, person starts eating a large quantity of it. Second reason is the burning of fewer calories after the stoppage of intake of nicotine. This may be justified by the fact that nicotine is responsible to higher the rate of burning calories, and when a person has suddenly stopped intake of nicotine, the calories burning process slows down, which ultimately leads to obesity. However, smoking is injurious to health and should be quitted to maintain the quality of life.

6.   Age

Age is yet another important factor that leads to obesity. Aging leads to the loss of muscles, especially when there is little activities in life. As a result, muscles loss leads to the decrease in the amount of burnt calories as the whole process is affected and decelerates. So, with the increase of age, if the calories intake is not reduced, the person may gain weight and develop obesity.

7.

Menopause and Pregnancy in Women

One of important reasons of weight gain in women is the menopause with age. Women normally gain 5pounds of weight at this stage and develop a dense fat layer around their waist.

Yet another important reason is the pregnancy in women. During pregnancy, usually women gain weight as the child is developing and this is the need for the child. But, after giving birth to the baby, they need to breast feed the baby and are unable to maintain their weight back to the normal weight. So, after a few pregnancies, usually women develop enough fats, and become obese.

8.   **Lack of Sleep**

Lack of sleep is also one of the potential causes of obesity as this habit makes person eat more high caloric food, which leads to the accumulation of fats in the body. Sleep helps to regulate a few of the important hormones, including ghrelin, leptin, and insulin. If these hormones are not properly regulated, a person may develop diabetes and obesity.

So, In a nutshell, weight gain can be evaded by taking precautionary measures, which include mostly the ways to evade these risk factors. To enjoy a proper healthy life, it is very important to monitor your weight to standard levels, hence you can live a happy natural life forever.

3. Why you Gain Weight and Importance of Ideal Body Type

Why Is A Slender Body Type Preferred?

Why is being skinny admirable? What are the benefits of having and maintaining a proper body mass? These are the questions that can be answered very easily with logic. Having a control of your weight ensures good health for the individual for present, and also while he ages on. Over the years, many people gain weight without even noticing, and before they realize they are overweight, become obese enough that they cannot find the right amount of time and energy to become slender again. Sticking to a healthy lifestyle and healthy food is important to avoid getting fat over time. Having a slender body is really good for the health. People having a normal body weight are at a reduced risk for many dangerous disease like diabetes, hypertension, cardiovascular problems, stroke, arthritis, gall stones, infertility, asthma, sleep apnea, snoring, cataracts etc. Slender body and normal body weight gives you a confidence about your body and appearance. Although, it is also important to feel confident about yourself irrespective of your body weight and physical appearance, but, it is also equally important to become of normal weight and feel even more positive about yourself.

What Causes Weight Gain- Calories in Vs Calories out

Weight gain is due to a very simple and interesting fact that the amount of weight gain is equal to the difference of calories intake and calories utilized.

Weight change = calories in − calories out

If you eat as much calories in a day as you burn, weight gain will be zero. But, if you eat more calories than you burn, they are deposited in your body, hence de-shaping your body and increasing your weight drastically.

Decreasing the quantity of food taken per day and shifting towards less processed foods helps with weight loss. Shifting towards a diet with more vegetables and fruits have a proven record in weight loss. The quantity of food in your diet is a major factor in deciding your obesity. Although

change in type of food is important, but eating a lot of quality food is also not recommended. Reducing quantity of food in general, be it healthy or unhealthy, is the key. By reducing the quantity of food in your everyday life, you are forcing your body to utilize the stored calories for routine bodily functions.

Some people tend to gain more weight as compared to others, even though they eat almost same quantities as others. This is because of some genetic predisposition to obesity, but it is not so severe that a little effort cannot mitigate it.

The second important decider in weight gain is lack of activity and lack of exercise. The less your body moves, the less calories it utilizes. Sitting makes you fatter than standing, while standing makes you fatter than walking, and so on. The more physical activity means the more consumption of calories up to the point when stored calories from body starts to consume by our body. Avoid watching a lot of television or sitting at a computer as this promotes little to no activity at all.

Third factor contributing in weight gain is the lack sleep. Researchers studied people on same diet with different sleeps concluded that people with less sleep tend to gain more weight.

4. How to Achieve and Maintain a Normal Body Weight- Countering Negativity and Losing Weight

There is no shortcut to achieving an ideal body weight. There is no magic food to reduce weight overnight. There is no magic exercise either. This doesn't mean it cannot be achieved. Achieving a healthy body weight is a combination of some lifestyle changes like moving towards healthy food, avoiding high carbohydrates food and doing regular physical activity. The more important thing is to keep a positive attitude that it quite possible with little practice.

Strategies to Evade Obesity and Weight Gain

Following are a few strategies by which you can counter the negativity in your life and achieve a perfect body shape that will make your personality stand out of the crowd.

Healthy Diet

Healthy diet is very important in trying to achieve a lower body weight. Some people believe the low carbohydrate diet works better than low fat diet. Actually it's the balance between two, both carbohydrates and fats needs to be reduced. The quantity of food also plays a key role. A lot of good food will still lead to gain in weight. So, to maintain a proper balance, the quantity of food needs to be reduced because they also give in calories to our body. Eating fewer calories is the main strategy under healthy diet. For starters, try to decrease at least 500 calories from your daily intake. The amount of a food being processed is also crucial. The more something is processed, makes it more unnatural and unhealthier to the body. For example, you will gain less weight eating peanuts than will gain while eating peanut butter. Eating whole grain is more beneficial than eating refined grain. Similarly, whole wheat should be preferred than eating refined wheat bread. Slow foods should be preferred to fast foods. Home cooked meals are much better than restaurants and specially fast foods. Decrease consumption of fast food to maximum two times per month.

Carbonated beverages are the most resilient factors in people gaining weight. The corporations have designed their sodas with formulas that are difficult to remove from our diet. A single Can of soda gives calories, which are consumed by 20 minutes of jogging, and it's a lot of calories. You must get rid of carbonated drinks for your diet plan to work. In my observation, keeping away from carbonated beverages for one continuous starting week is difficult, and after one week, you will not feel the need to drink them. Consider switching to water instead of soda, or if much desired have a fresh fruit juice instead of soda. Remember, Soda is your enemy.

Increase Intake of Water

Researchers in Germany reported that water consumption increases the rate at which our body burn calories. The procedure requires an adequate supply of water in order to function efficiently and dehydration slows down the fat-burning process. Burning calories creates toxins, which are removed out of our body with the help of water. Water helps maintain muscle tone by assisting muscles to contract, hence are very useful in lubricating your joints. It is also believed that appropriate hydration can help reduce muscle and joint soreness when exercising. Drinking plenty of water is recommended.

Alcohol
Alcohol should be used only moderately. Excess alcohol intake have very negative effects on weight loss. Our body uses alcohol as its fuel and burns alcohol instead of other carbohydrates Alcohol should be used only moderately. Excess alcohol intake have very negative effects on weight loss. Our body uses alcohol as its fuel and burns alcohol instead of other carbohydrates and fats. Therefore, the body is ended up storing carbohydrates and fats from diet in body and burning the alcohol.

By countering all these negativity from your life, eventually, you will choose a healthy and happy life for yourself.

5. Meal Plan for Weight Loss- Things That Can Wreck Your Weight Loss Dreams

There is no ideal meal plan that each and every person trying to lose weight must adapt. There are certain foods that can be avoided to reduce calories intake. Moreover, there are certain foods that help increase the metabolism rate (the process by which food is burnt in our body is called metabolism).

For a general overview of a simple meal plan while following the other instructions, consider the following. Also these are among the foods that speeds up your metabolism, hence leaving you lean.

1.

Fruits and Vegetables

The best thing about vegetables and fruits is that they are densely loaded with nutrients, but not densely loaded with calories. So, it is recommended to add a lot of different natural colors to your food, and by colors, we mean fresh fruits and vegetables of different colors. Most of the fruits and vegetables are good for health in terms of weight loss as compared to other foods, but obviously, some are more beneficial. We recommend you to add spinach, carrots, cranberries, pineapple, blueberries, kale and celery to your weight loss diet.

2.

Whole Foods

Whole foods are unprocessed and unrefined foods, or they are refined and processed as little as possible, before being consumed. Whole foods usually do not contain fats, carbohydrates or added salt. Whole foods includes but are not limited to unpolished grains, beans, vegetables, fruits and other products comprising non-homogenized dairy products and meat. Using a whole food product means maximum utilization of natural constituents of the food with almost no detrimental effects on the body. Eating whole foods helps prevents diseases. They are most near to natural state and therefore provides a range of helpful nutrients.

It is difficult to start consuming whole foods completely in our diet because of modern era lifestyle, but it is possible to make a good 60-70 percent of our diet from whole foods.

Whole foods includes:

- Unprocessed fruits and vegetables.
- Beans & Legumes including kidney beans, chickpeas and lentils.
- Whole grains, including oats, buckwheat, brown rice, rye, whole wheat, millet, quinoa and cornmeal.
- Seeds and nuts.
- Animal origin whole foods includes eggs, small whole fish, seafood, poultry and red meat, such as lamb, beef and veal.

3.

Breakfast

Remove instant oatmeal, boxed cereals, commercial pastries and muffins from your breakfast menus and shift to a more natural and whole foods based one. Use an omelet with spinach, tomatoes and mushrooms or use full fat plain yogurt made from natural milk.

4.

Lunch and Dinner

Include more vegetables and proteins to your lunch and dinner. Use an additional salad made from lettuce, cabbage, onions, tomatoes, avocado and olive oil. Use only cold pressed oils because it is a very basic process in the extraction of oil. A variety of meals can be prepared by the use of various seasoning and spices like parsley, turmeric, basil, cumin or chili powder in different vegetables, proteins and fats. The thought and effort you put into making your food counts, because it is giving importance to your decision of healthy diet.

5.   **Desserts**

As the whole foods meals are rich with nutrients and very resourceful, mostly a need to have dessert is diminished, but occasionally, desserts can be taken. A healthy dessert can be a fruit salad e.g. made with berries or avocado. You can use cocoa powder on mashed avocado for dessert without hurting your body by loading it with unhealthy foods.

6.   Snacks

Most of the snack foods available to us are processed foods and have almost no nutritional value. Foods like potato chips, granola bars, mochas, chocolates, energy drinks and carbonated beverages are the first line snacks available in our society, and all of these are unhealthy and should be replaced by healthy alternatives. Consuming these foods as snacks can lead to even more hunger over time and consequent consumption of more food thus making a vicious cycle making you gain more weight. Healthy alternative snacks can be some dried fruits nuts like almonds, pistachios, cashew nuts, beef jerky or even a boiled egg. Of course fruits like banana, oranges or apples can be very healthy form of snacks.

Avoid packaged foods, as these have been processed and are void of nutritional value. Foods that have a longer shelf life or expiry means they are even void of nutrition.

7.	**Tea**

Green tea is the healthiest beverage on the planet. It's almost unbelievable how much beneficial green tea is. It has almost a hundred benefits. You should include a few cups of little sweetened green tea to your daily routine. It helps in burning fats, and yet, along with physical activity in the form of exercise, green tea helps to burn body fats a little faster. Green tea increase the metabolic rate, thus increasing fat burning and enhancing energy expenditure. Making green tea a routine drink in your day can be more beneficial for you in your weight loss target. It can be used as hot beverage or taken as a cold tea with ice and a little added lime or lemon grass for additional flavoring. Some other herbal teas, specifically made for slimming can also be used, but just plain green tea is what we recommend. It is also available in many flavors for change of taste like jasmine. Green tea is one of the potential enhancers of metabolism in your body, hence leaving you lean. You can carry a sealed tea bag in pocket anywhere you like. You can also add it to your normal coffee.

6. Physical Activity- A Key to Success

There is no denial that exercise is one of most crucial part of losing weight. There is no other method following which exercise can be "bypassed". In order to remain healthy and to maintain a healthy physique, you have to stay active. If you are not using your muscles, eventually you will lose them and let your body be dominated by fats.

Whatever exercise you choose to do, the key is doing it regularly. Make physical activity an inevitable part of your daily routine. No matter what happens in your day, you have to do that exercise on a daily basis, just like you have to go to bathroom every day. What specific set of exercise to do is more relevant to the body type and weight, but, generally a few routines can help most of the individuals looking to get slim and lose some extra pounds. Regular physical activity helps to maintain a healthy body. It helps to

keep dangerous diseases away. It helps to strengthen your muscles, joints and bones. It helps to condition heart and lungs. It helps in building overall strength and improves your sleep. Moreover, it increases your self-esteem, prevents depression and relieves stress.

Walking

It is recommended to have a brisk walk for minimum 30-45 minutes daily, and have it increased as much as possible after a few days of practice. At brisk pace, a walk for 30 minutes will cover 1.5 to 2 miles. The following guide can be used as a reference to weight loss by walking.

- For the starting 5-8 minutes, walk with an easy pace as a warm up.
- After warm up, do stretching and flexibility exercises.
- Walk for next 30-60 minutes at a brisk pace.
- Slow down and walk at a slower pace for 5 minutes.
- Some easy stretching at the end of walk.

If you can walk more time, it is more beneficial. Don't limit to the above mentioned time of 30-45 minutes because the more, the better. Walking on treadmill or outdoors in park or a playground is equally recommended. If outdoor environment can give you more fresh air, then it is recommended to walk outside. On an estimated average, walking on a brisk pace for 30 minutes will burn about 150 calories. Burning 500 calories per day leads to losing a pound per week. For starters, start with easy routine with a day off in the first week. After you get used to, and your body picks your motivation for physical activity, you can increase your time and pace as suited for you. Develop a routine of regular exercise because its importance is not decreased even after you reduce your weight. Studies have shown that, to maintain a lower weight after weight loss, regular exercise is mandatory. Don't look at it as a burden because once you get to a routine with it, you will actually enjoy it. It's a healthy lifestyle with lots of positive energy.

Add hills, slopes and stairs to your walking routes. Walking uphill burns far more calories than a normal plain route. Similarly, walking on stairs burns more calories, in fact, 4 more calories per minute.

Losing weight by walking is burning calories one by one, so, it is important to decrease calories intake also, especially sweets, candies, chocolates, cakes and confectioneries etc. Eating less is the key to weight loss by walking.

Running and Jogging

Running is considered as one of the most efficient means of burning body fat. Instead of running for fast pace and little time, consider running for longer duration of time with nominal pace. Simply, this can be put as *"To lose more weight, you have to give more time"*. One mistake people make with running is that they start consuming more beverages and it leads to intake of more calories and running seems useless for weight loss. Water is a healthy alternative to normal sugar containing beverages. Consider green tea if something else is desired other than water. As with walking, a regular routine is to be followed with only a day off from running if required. It's better to write down the complete schedule of running for the week and tick off the days that you followed your routine. This type of checking off the days you ran is also a type of self-motivation. Next week, carry on this routine in reverse so that your body does not adapt to the routine because if you do the same routine again and again, then your body adapts to it and you end up burning fewer calories. Try to change the loops and tracks where you run so that your body face a constant changing running environment.

Push ups
It's a false perception that pushups are only the upper arm exercise. It is actually general body strengthening exercise with positive effects on arms, pectorals, chest, abdomen, diaphragm, torso and even thighs. By stimulating a lot of muscles during pushups, our body needs a lot of energy, which is provided by burning of fats and carbohydrates. Pushups helps a lot in development of general body shape.

Negativity Surrounding Weight Loss
Although the start of a weight loss ritual is very energetic and motivating. It gives us hope, which helps us keep moving forward. But, after sometime, a lot of people become pessimist and lose hope instead of losing weight. There are certain things to keep in mind in order to avoid getting into such a situation. At the start of weight loss routine, note down your weight and even BMI on a notebook or in your computer with date. Don't use the weighing scale for a complete month. No matter how tempting it may be to check your weight after that tough exercise you just made, don't do it. After following the basic diet plan and various physical activity routines for at least one month, you can measure your weight again and you will not be disappointed. Write this down again with date and then start your next month. It is customary to mention here that it is not all about weight and scale. Some people may lose very little weight on scale, but will

seem to lose some physically. This is because the body loses fats and carbohydrates and develops some muscles and bones also. So, even though you might seem to lose less weight, you will still be going towards an attractive and slender physique. In such conditions, when weight loss is not much on the scale but still physical body measurements like waist circumference, chest size, bra size and shape of the buttocks will change.

How to Monitor Your Weight
A weighing scale may give you a different reading at different time of the day. This is because our body faces some changes over the period of day. Some factors contributing to this variation are water, food and clothes. The correct method is weighting yourself in the morning after waking up and before the breakfast. Take reading for two consecutive days and calculate its average as your default weight. After following your diet and exercise plan for a month, weigh again for two consecutive days in the morning in the same manner and use the average. Also measure the circumference of your waist, just around belly button, and around the mid of buttocks using a soft measuring tape. Do not monitor your weight every day because such measurements leads to negativity and might lead you into thinking that your efforts are not very fruitful.

Conclusion

Losing weight is something that a lot of us aspire. It is not an instant process with immediate results. Weight loss is a slow process, but, it is very fruitful. By following some easy but adaptable rules in our day to day life, we can manage to achieve weight loss and wow others and ourselves. Weight loss needs commitment and motivation, and also some optimism. Proper changes made to diet can lead to a correction in the calories input and utilization ratio, leading to burning of body fats. Proper food can also increase body energy, strength and attractiveness. Physical activity is also an integral part of weight loss. It is equally important to be strong and fit as it is to be slender. Exercise have a bundle of positive impacts on our bodies, including health improvement and weight loss. In order to be successful in losing weight, one must be motivated with optimist. Losing weight is very much possible, but it requires following some guidelines and making healthy changes in lifestyle.

Lose weight and Stay Awesome

Some of my other Workout/Recipe Books are listed below:
Book1
Book2
Book3
www.losingbellyfatmission.com
www.achieveitforyou.com

www.ingramcontent.com/pod-product-compliance
Lightning Source LLC
Chambersburg PA
CBHW030540290526
45786CB00004B/1789